To my dearest Braylon, Mommy loves you very much

This is for you & all the other children who have food allergies

May you be strong, fearless & enjoy life to the fullest

Even though you're different, remember you're special.

-LM

Patty's Secret © 2013

Written by Leneille Moon

Illustrations by Brandon Fall, www.fallillustration.com

Copyright © Leneille Moon.

All rights reserved.

EpiPen® is a registered trademark of Mylan Inc. licensed exclusively

to its wholly-owned subsidiary, Mylan Specialty L.P.

Summary: This book is about Patty a girl that is just like everyone else but she has a huge secret she'd like to keep from her classmates on the first day of school. She has a twin brother that is almost just alike but they have one thing that's different. One thing that Patty doesn't want to share with her new friends. What do you think it is?

Library of Congress Control Number: 2013909103

ISBN: 978-1475189490

Patty's Secret

A Tale of a Girl with Food Allergies

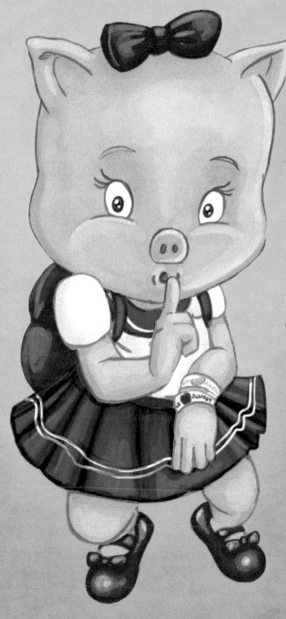

Written by Leneille Moon

Illustrated by Brandon Fall

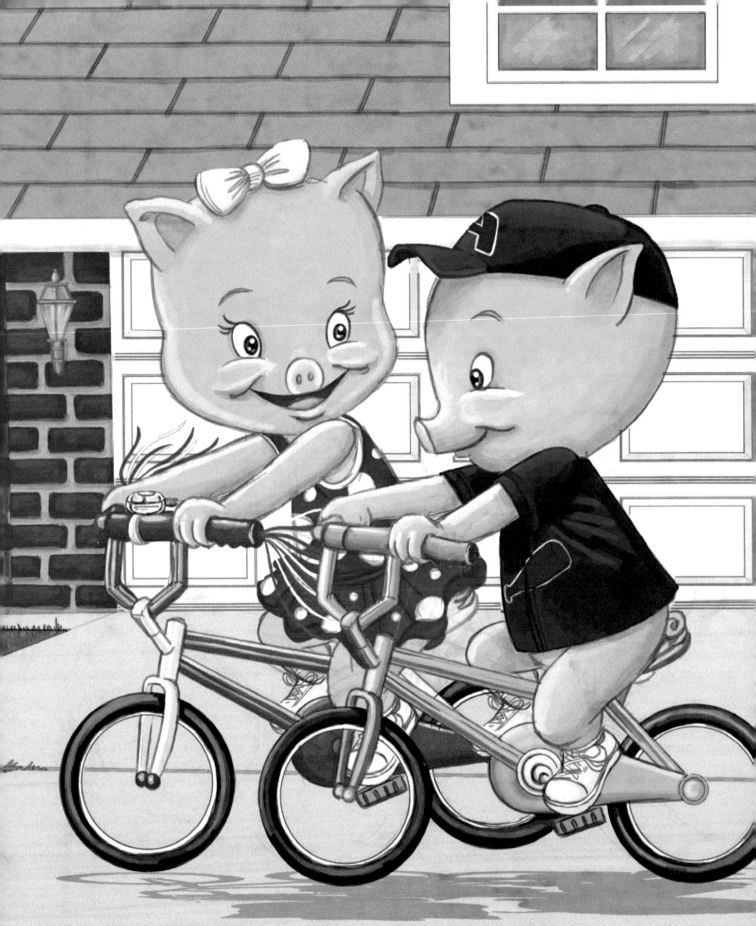

Patty and Patrick are twin pigs. They like to do everything together. They ride bikes together, they play in the water fountain together, and they even love to pop bubbles together.

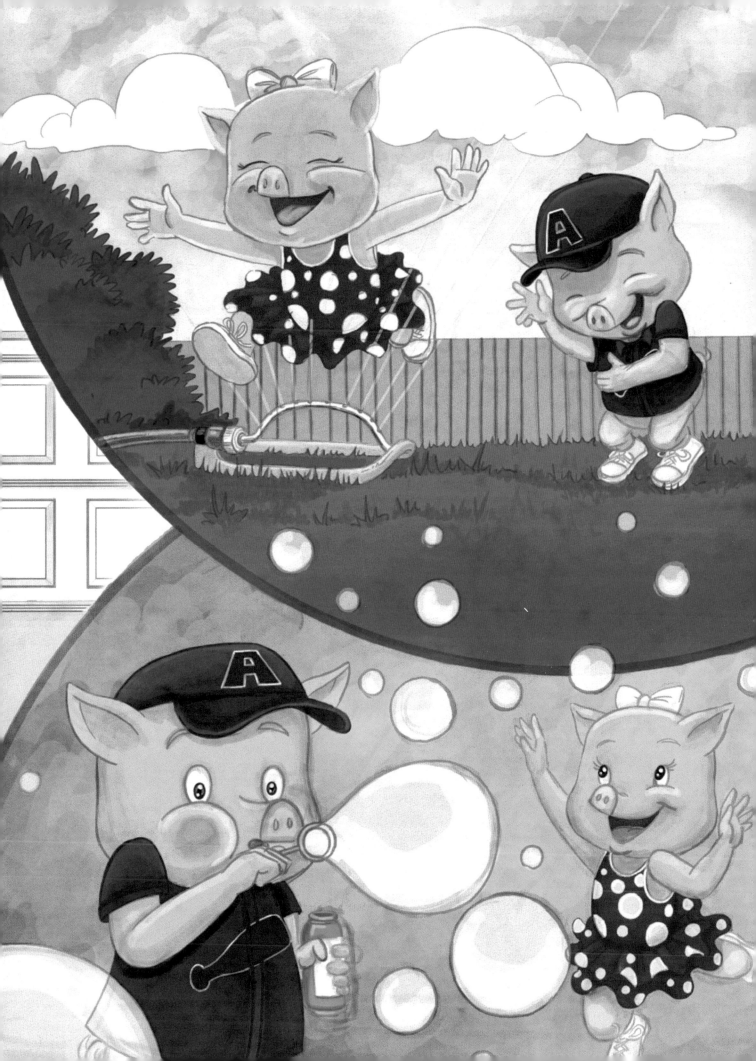

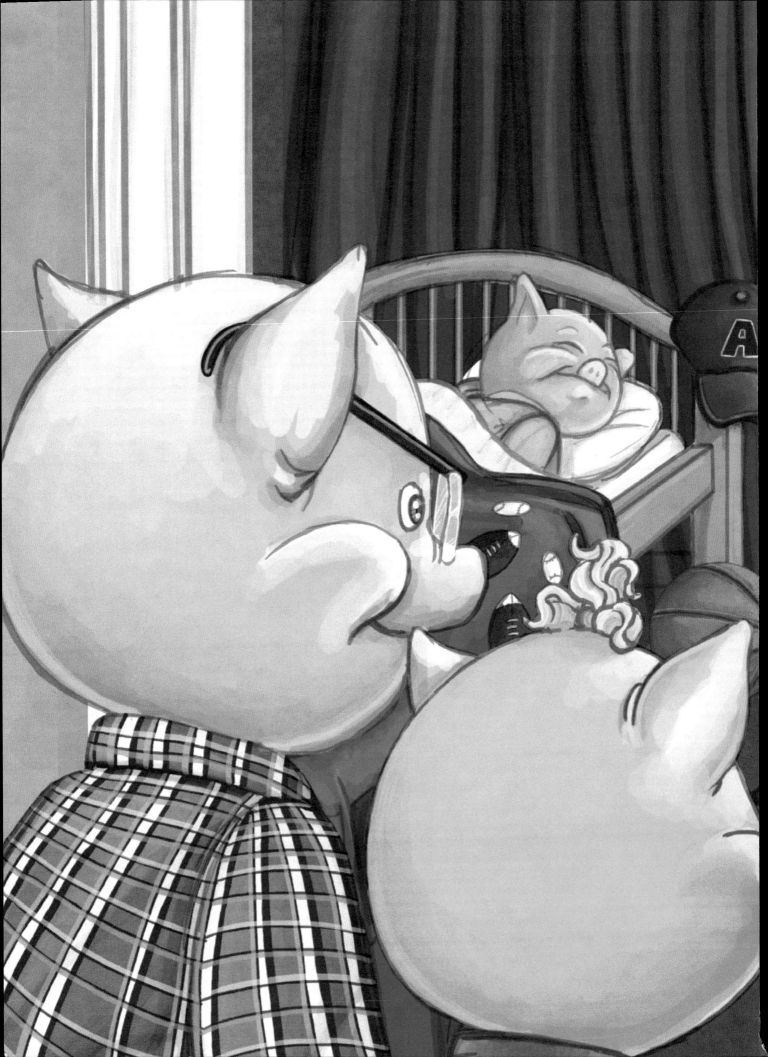

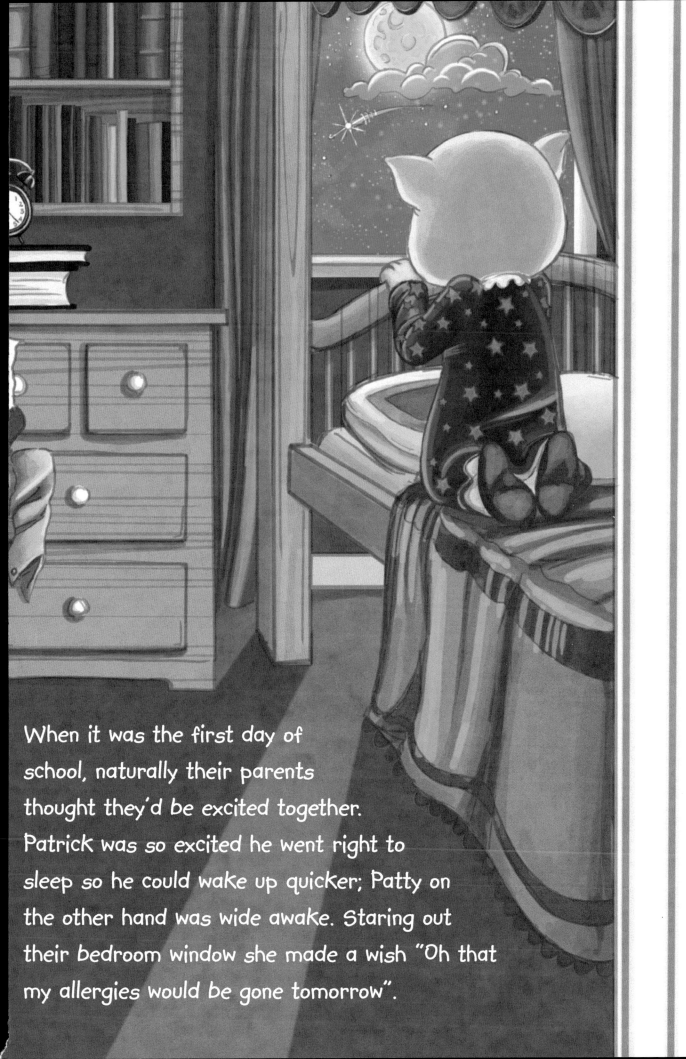

When it was the first day of
school, naturally their parents
thought they'd be excited together.
Patrick was so excited he went right to
sleep so he could wake up quicker; Patty on
the other hand was wide awake. Staring out
their bedroom window she made a wish "Oh that
my allergies would be gone tomorrow".

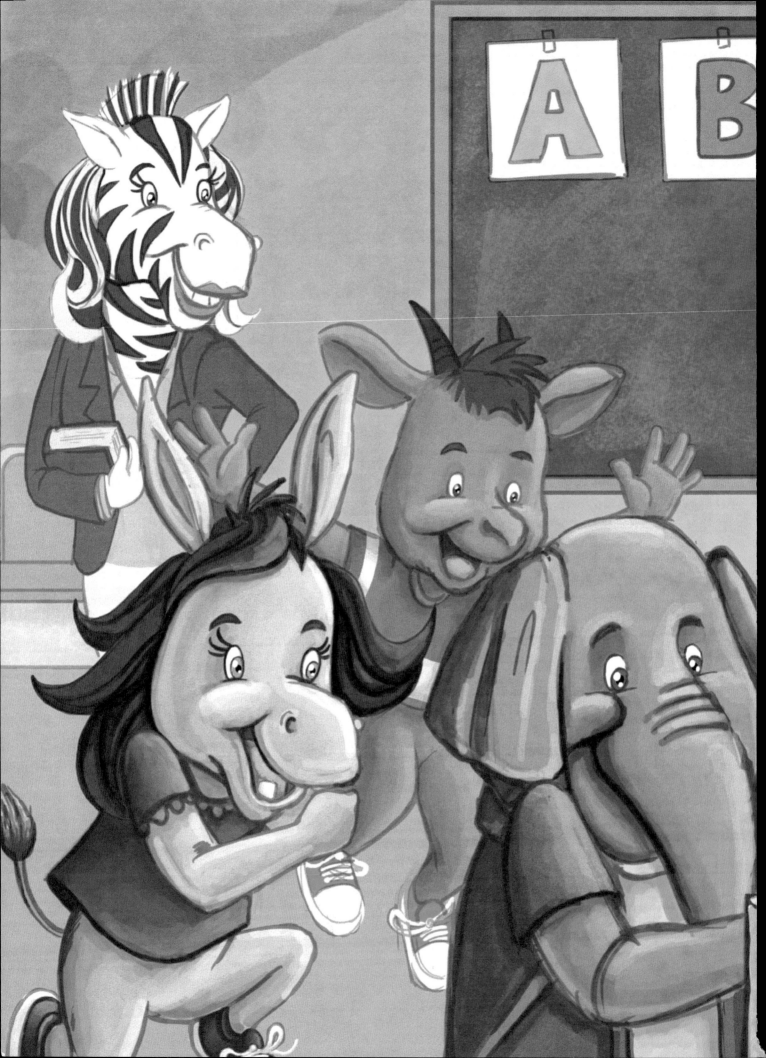

Off they went Monday morning onto the school bus and into Mrs. Zebra's classroom. The children laughed and played all day until the bell rang for lunch.

"Oh dear" said Patty as all the other children ran to their cubby to get their lunch boxes for lunch

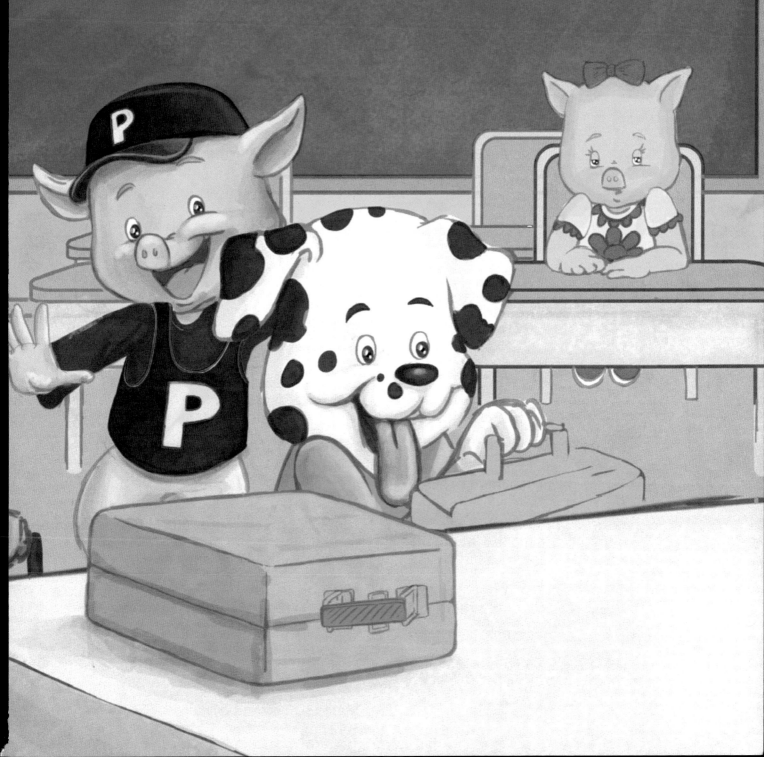

There were all kinds of lunchboxes, there was a big purple butterfly one, the green dinosaur one and Patrick's was a red fire truck... Patty had a pink floral pail with bright stickers with everything she's allergic to.

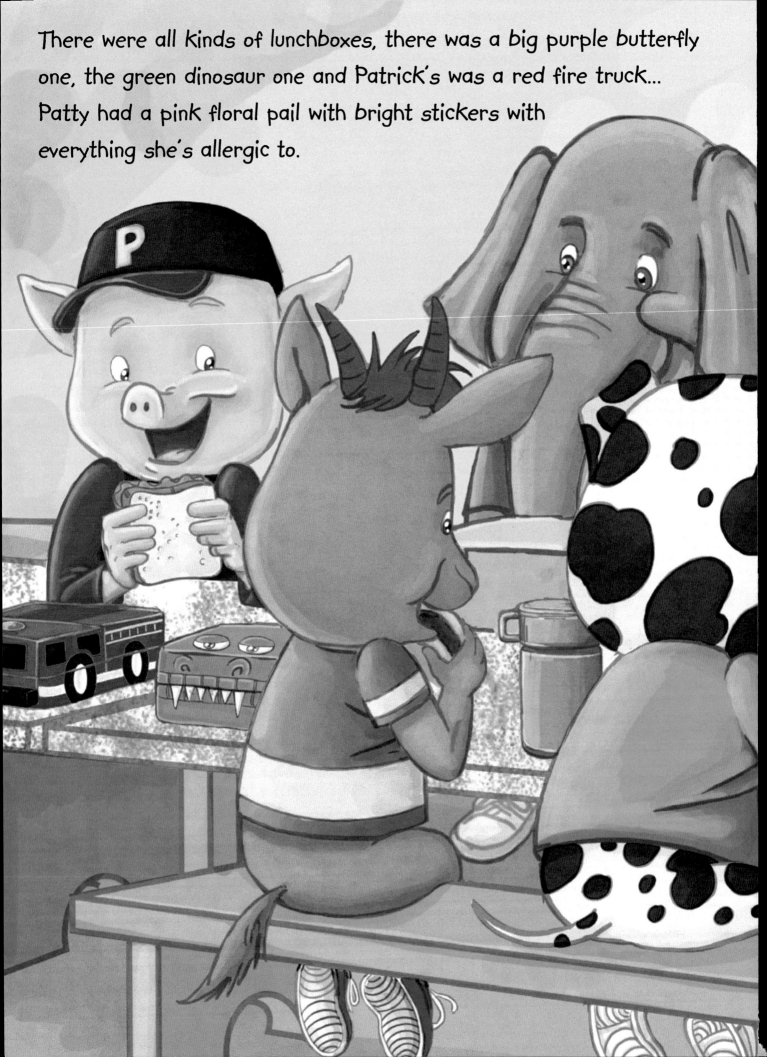

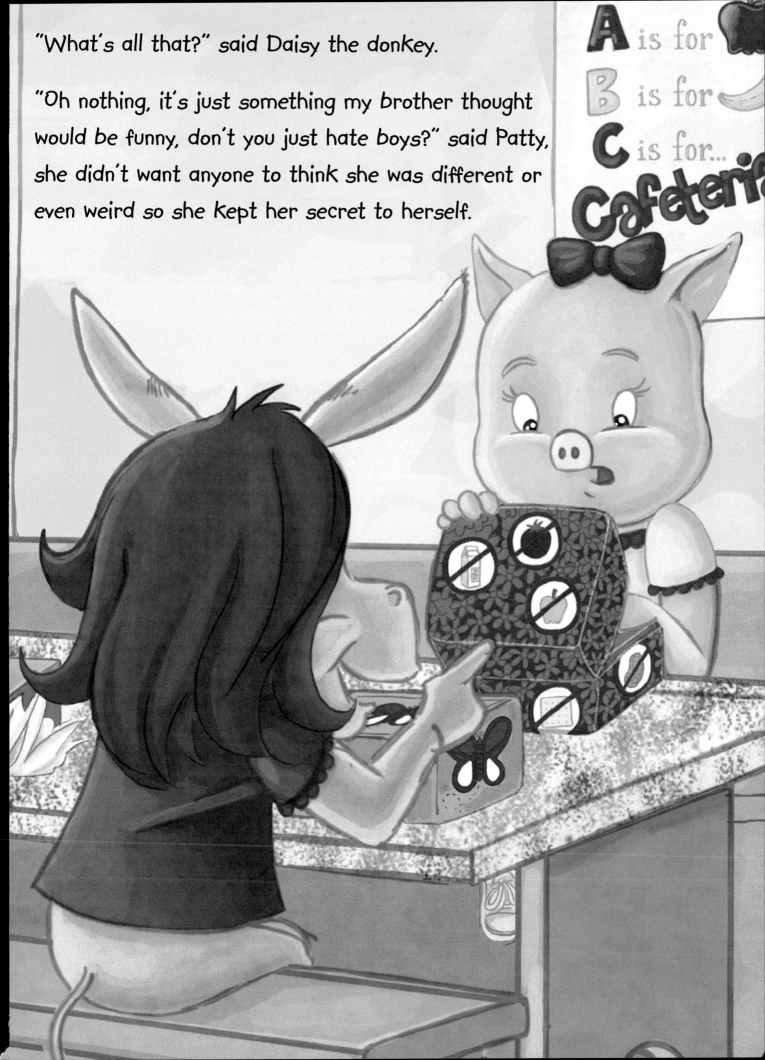

"What's all that?" said Daisy the donkey.

"Oh nothing, it's just something my brother thought would be funny, don't you just hate boys?" said Patty, she didn't want anyone to think she was different or even weird so she kept her secret to herself.

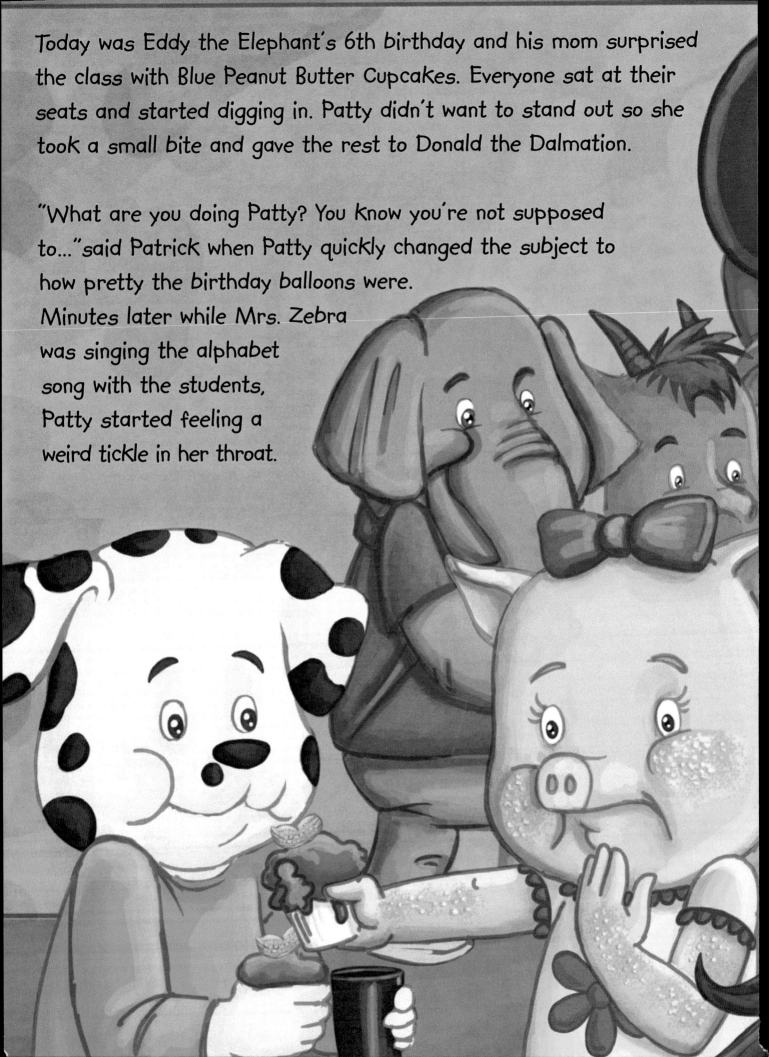

Today was Eddy the Elephant's 6th birthday and his mom surprised the class with Blue Peanut Butter Cupcakes. Everyone sat at their seats and started digging in. Patty didn't want to stand out so she took a small bite and gave the rest to Donald the Dalmation.

"What are you doing Patty? You know you're not supposed to..."said Patrick when Patty quickly changed the subject to how pretty the birthday balloons were.
Minutes later while Mrs. Zebra was singing the alphabet song with the students, Patty started feeling a weird tickle in her throat.

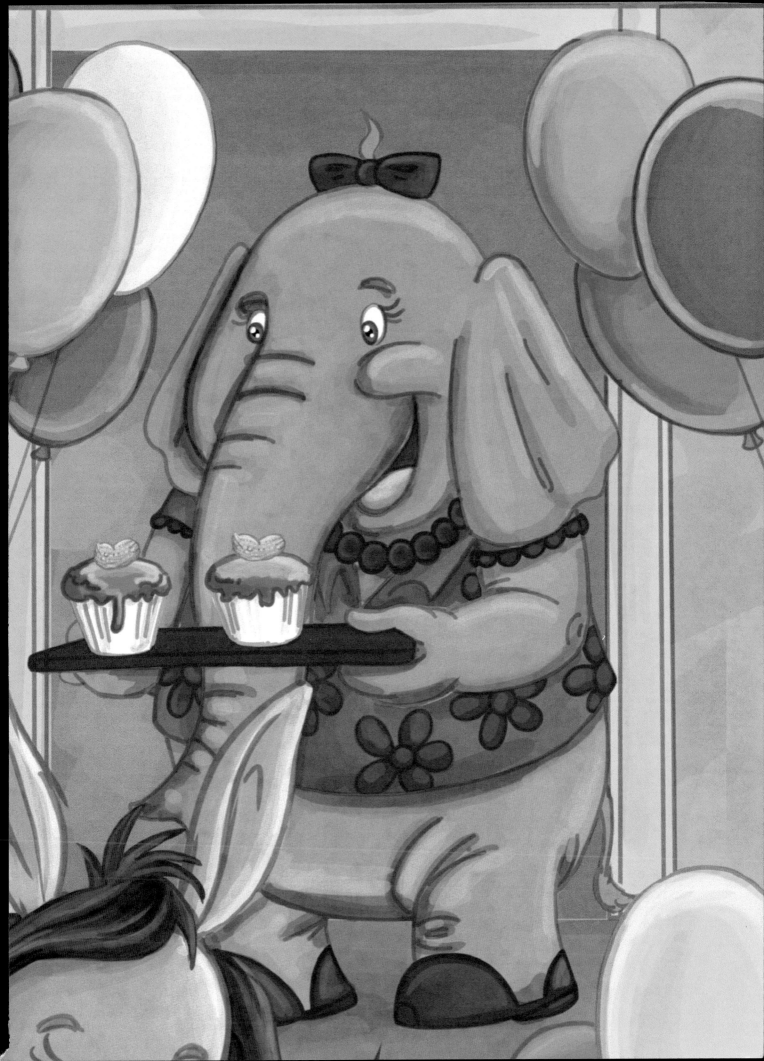

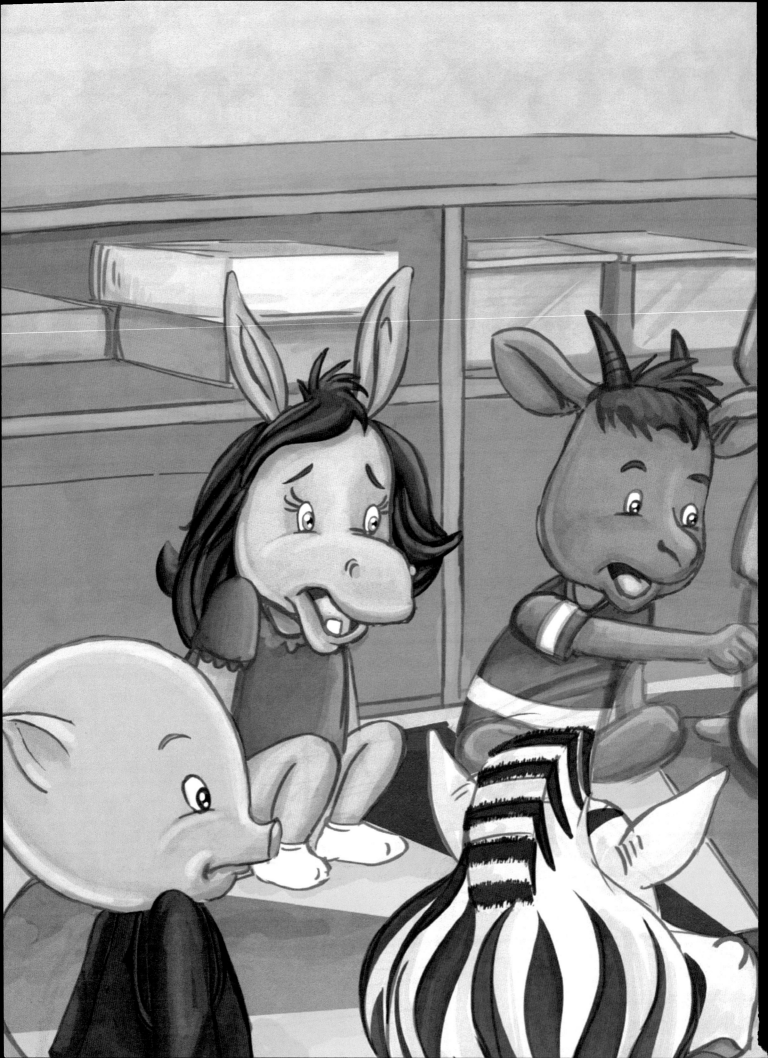

Patty coughed and continued singing. Little did she know that her cheek had turned apple red and her left eye was beginning to swell shut. "Paaaattttttyyyyy!!!" Gabby the Goat yelled. All the children began staring and pointing at Patty's face. Patty was totally embarrassed.

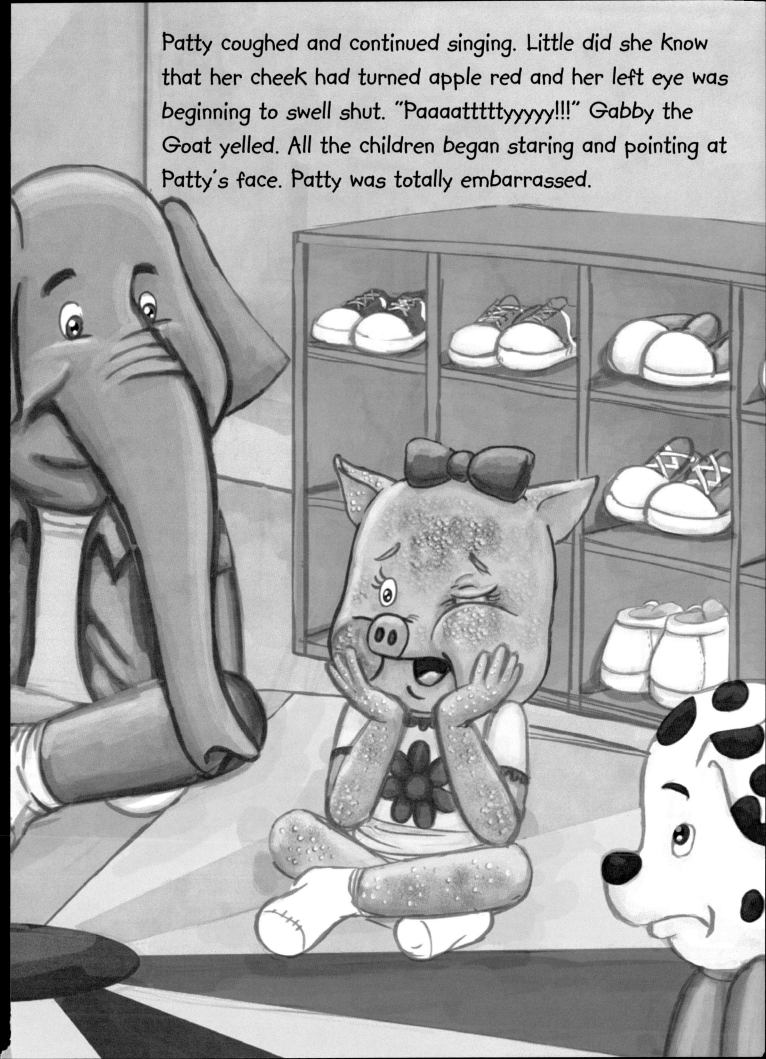

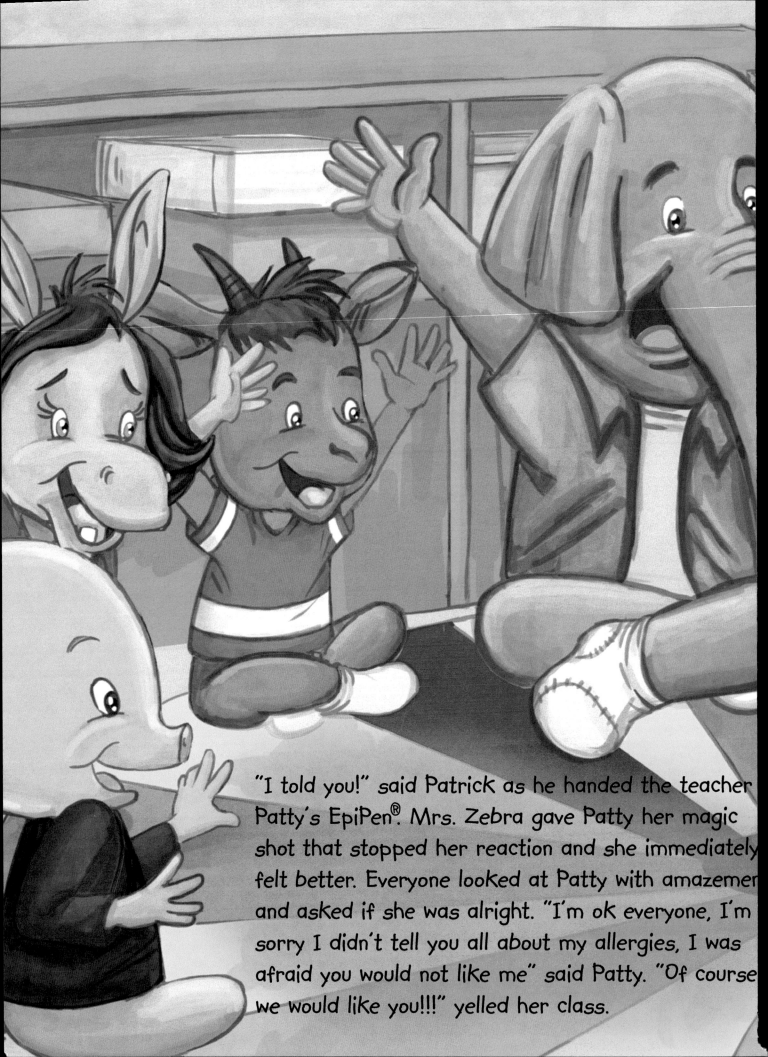

"I told you!" said Patrick as he handed the teacher Patty's EpiPen®. Mrs. Zebra gave Patty her magic shot that stopped her reaction and she immediately felt better. Everyone looked at Patty with amazement and asked if she was alright. "I'm ok everyone, I'm sorry I didn't tell you all about my allergies, I was afraid you would not like me" said Patty. "Of course we would like you!!!" yelled her class.

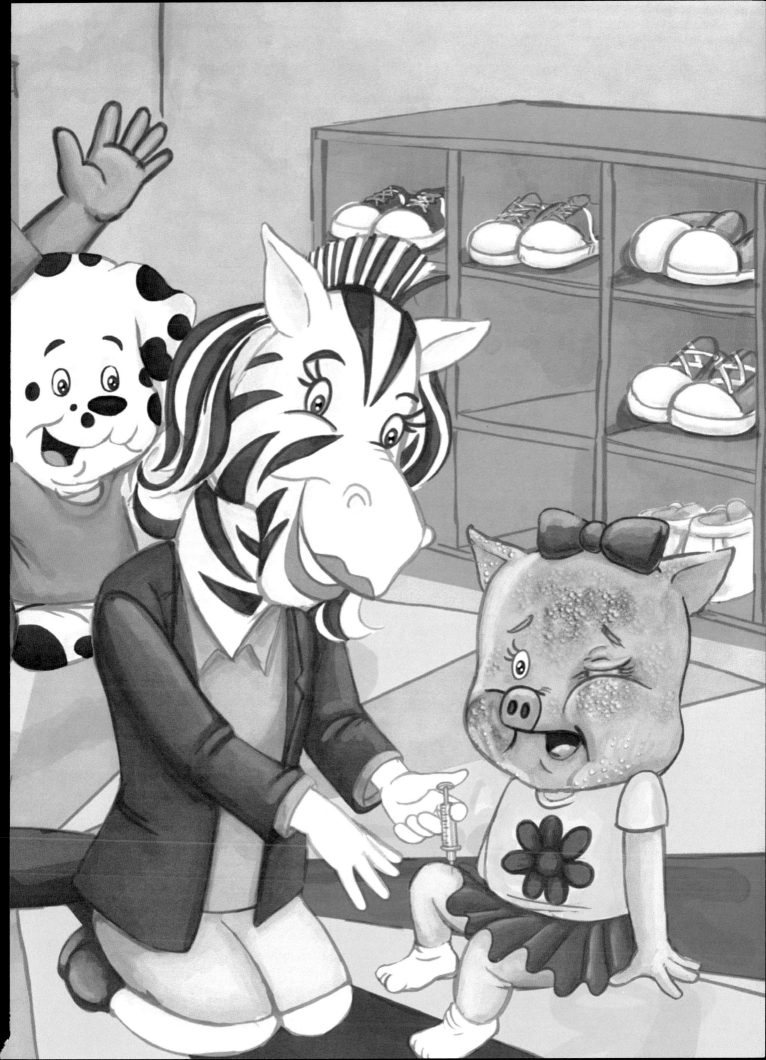

"My sister is awesome, she just can't eat nuts, milk or eggs, but she's just like all of us" said Patrick.

"That's right" said Mrs. Zebra, "there's nothing to be afraid of Patty, but it's important that you tell everyone about your allergies so that this does not happen again".

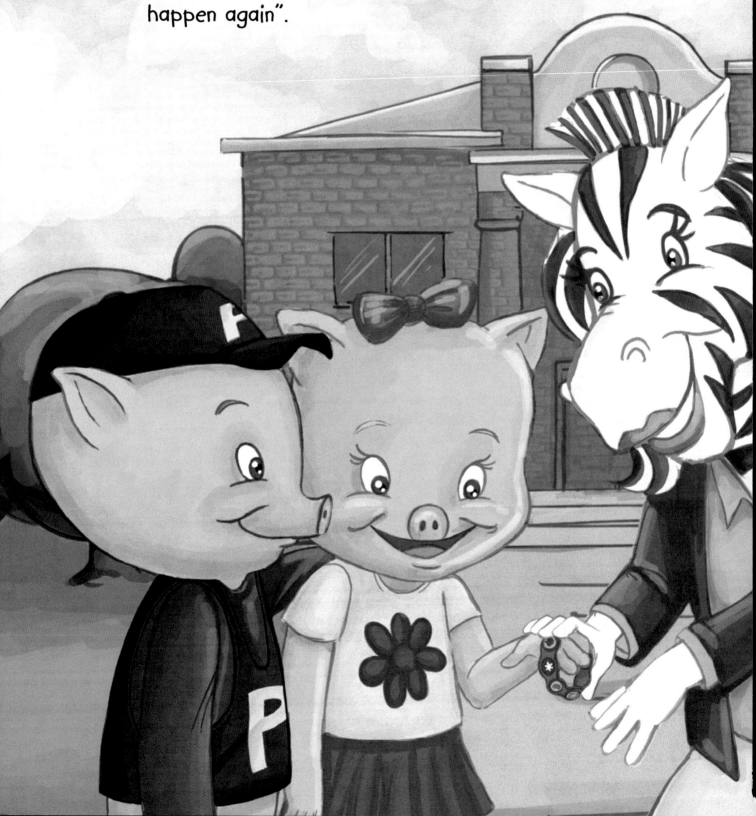

She gave Patty a special bracelet to put on her wrist. It listed all her allergies so she would never forget to tell her friends.

Patty learned that day that her allergies were not a curse but a challenge and she could be healthy and safe as long as she didn't hide the truth.

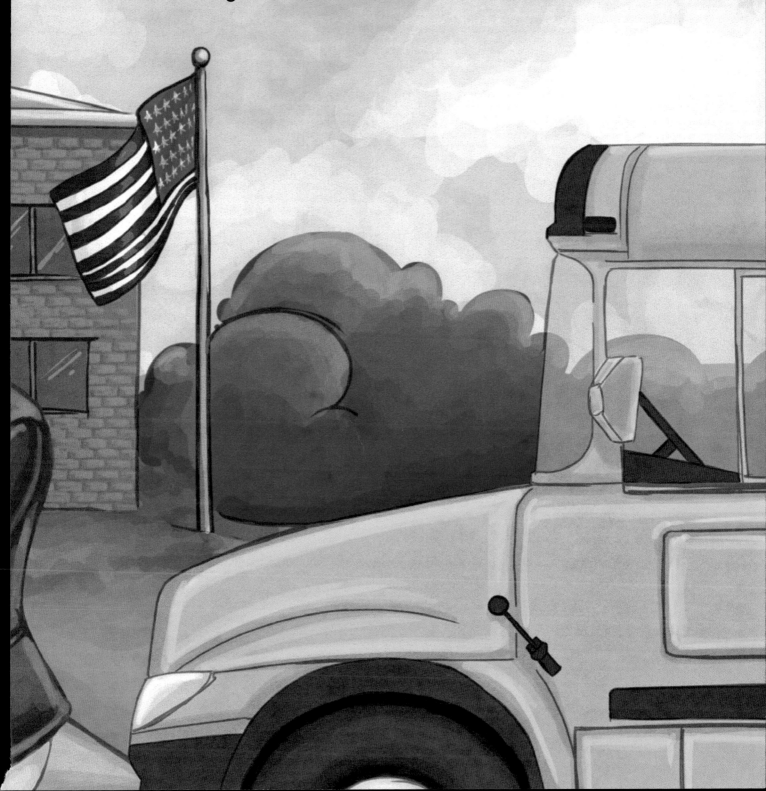

Food Allergy Word Search

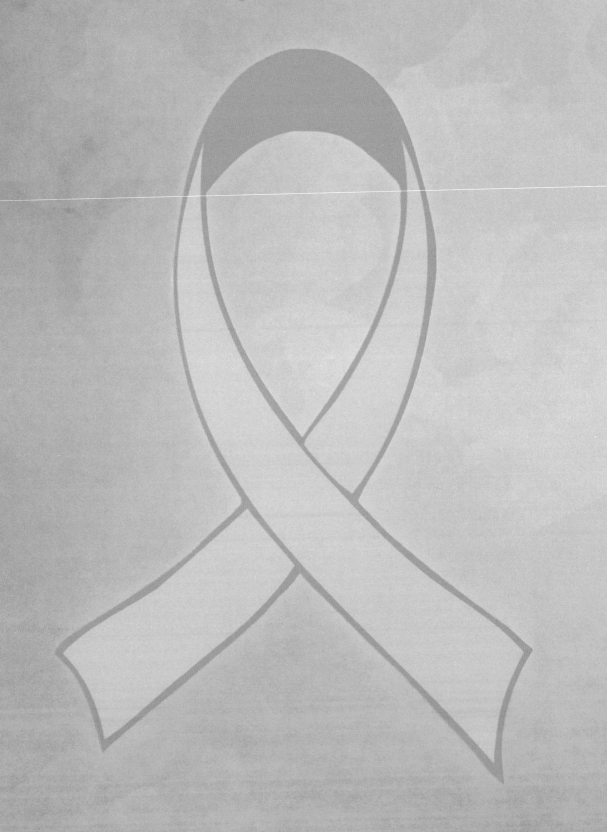

a b x s x t t r h e
d w r k c r w s k p
t u n a e p i r l i
t e l e c f w s i p
w a n i l e g x m e
d u e l r g l k n n
t v e h e x x e t l
o h a r w s o y t d
s a l l e r g i s t
f u y q g n r z q c

---

allergist	peanut
bracelet	shellfish
eggs	soy
EpiPen®	treenut
milk	wheat

Food Allergy Facts (According to FARE-Food Allergy Research and Education):
Did you know Food Allergies affects 1 in every 13 children (under 18 years of age) in the U.S. That's about two in every classroom.

The top 8 Allergens are: Milk, Wheat, Eggs, Peanuts, Treenuts, Soy, Shellfish and Fish.

Kids with food allergies look like me and you, they aren't a specific race, gender or neighborhood, they are from every walk of life and the people around them have a very tough task of managing their food allergies by reading ingredients, washing their hands not to spread the allergens around and remembering to always carry their EpiPen®.

To find out more about kids
with food allergies
ask an adult to visit:

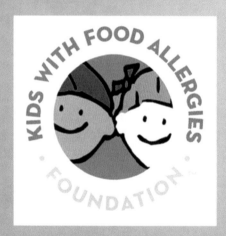

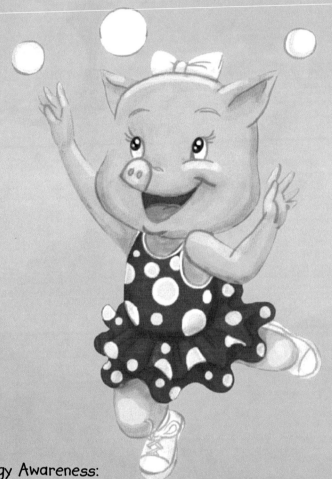

Kidswithfoodallergies.org

Ways you can support Food Allergy Awareness:
1. Purchase food allergy children's books
   like this one and donate it to a local library
2. Read this book to your class
3. Donate to Food Allergy Organization in your town or nationally
4. Support & Uplift your kids with food allergies to deter bullying

Visit FAKidsatl.org to find out how you can help spread the word to your friends, family or classmates about food allergy awareness.